The UK
Slow Cooker
Recipe Book

Quick, Nutritious Meals for Everyone
incl. Vegan and Vegetarian Bonus

[1st Edition]

Nathan James

ISBN – 9781712409190

Table of contents

Introduction

Once you've known cooking with a slow cooker, you can never go back. You have been warned. Convenience, time saving, and nutrition in one simple to use, easy to maintain, energy efficient little kitchen appliance.

It is always good to understand the appliance before using it. What is a slow cooker, then? This marvel of the kitchen has three basic constituents: The outer casing, the stoneware inner container, and the lid.

The metal casing houses the low-wattage heating coils and has the job of actually cooking the food.

The inner ceramic container lies snugly inside the metal casing. Most slow cookers allow for the removal of this inner pot.

Thirdly is the domed lid which tightly fits onto the inner ceramic pot.

Feel free to use cheap cuts with this forgiving cooking style. Because meal preparation is slow, even tougher meat cuts are cooked to tender perfection. Perfect for meals in a busy household. Simply toss in the Ingredients: and leave the cooker to cook while you get on with your life.

Tips

Choose the right temperature. Cooking times on HIGH are slightly longer than on LOW.

Dried herbs are better than fresh herbs in this long cooking process and will release flavour over time rather than wilt like the fresh certainly will.

On the point of herbs, fresh herbs should be added only towards the end of the cooking process to avoid them disappearing entirely and having no impact in the taste of the meal.

Forgiving as the slow cooker process is, do NOT lift the lid unnecessarily during cooking. The cooking time will be significantly increased by the heat lost during this act.

Frozen food can be used in the slow cooker, using all the necessary and due diligence only. Of course it will lead to an increased cooking time, and more importantly using frozen meat may increase the risk of food poisoning. Thawing is preferable....

Never leave food to cool in the cooker. Slow Cooker leftovers are perfect for refrigerating for another time, but they should always be cooled in a clean, appropriate container first. Food cooled and stored in the cooker are at risk of bacteria which is not what you will be wanting to serve up.

Cleaning the Slow Cooker

Many of the recipes for slow cookers involve only the slow cooker. This means only one pot to clean! The removable pot is ideal. Simply remove it, fill with soapy hot water and let it soak. Dry it and pack it away for the next time.

Before immersing in the cleaning of slow cookers, bear in mind that the instructions for your particular slow cooker must first and foremost be followed! All slow cookers are not equal, and this applies as much to the cleaning thereof as to the size and its cooking ability.

Never be tempted to clean the slow cooker until you have unplugged it. Never!

You can also make the cleaning process easier before you even start to cook. Greasing the slow cooker simply simplifies the imminent clean-up. Another convenient little effort and time saver is the slow cooker liner. This liner could feasibly also extend the usefulness and lifespan of the inner surface of your beloved slow cooker. Save time and effort with the use of a convenient cooking spray or a slow cooker liner.

Tough cooked in food will require a little more elbow grease. Simply fill the stoneware pot with water and cook the food off over a few hours on low temperature. You can even pop most stoneware slow cooker pots into the dishwasher. But ONLY the stoneware inserts, mind you. NEVER the outer casing which houses the electricals!

Not so easy is the cleaning of the exterior of the slow cooker or the interior of the slow cooker itself. Start with wiping it down with a soft cloth, wet through with warm soapy water. Avoid anything harsher than a mild detergent to make sure you are not damaging either the surface or its working parts. If the mild approach has not gleaned satisfactory results, try a cleaner specifically designed for the surface. A stainless-steel cleaner, for example. A baking soda and water mixture is usually a safe alternative which does a good job.

The underneath is quite often forgotten when cleaning. Spills and messes do reach the bottom of the slow cooker and must be cleaned. The area under the removable cooker houses the heating element and electrics and should not be submerged under water under any circumstances. Always make sure to cool this before cleaning.

You might want to take the removable parts off once every so often to give the slow cooker a thorough cleaning. Detachable handles and knobs will do with a good cleaning and should then be reassembled when dry.

Important Note

Braise tougher cuts to transform them into succulent, flavourful meals through the slow and lengthy application of moist heat at low temperature.

Brown certain cuts of meat beforehand, such as beef chuck, short ribs, pork shoulder, and spare ribs.

A good rule of thumb is to not fill the slow cooker pot by more than two-thirds.

Add dairy products last to avoid pools of oil or grainy residues.

Layering is imperative. The heat emanates from the bottom, and so it leads that foods at the base will cook before those towards the top of the cooker. Meats and root vegetables should therefore be closer to the heating element.

Prepare healthier meals, simply with these recipes which seldom call for fats or oils. Simmering in its own juices preserves vitamins and minerals which are typically lost during other cooking procedures.

Stewing in its own juices for long periods results in increased tenderizing and ultimate flavor, with nothing lost to evaporation or discarding of cooking liquids.

When cooking dishes which will not benefit from the added moisture of dripped liquids, lining the lid is the answer. Simply line the lid with paper towels on the inside. In this way liquid condensing on the cooker lid will not drip back into the food while cooking.

RECIPES

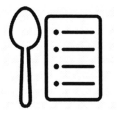

BREAKFAST

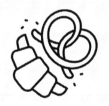

Breakfast Casserole

Time: 6hrs 20 minutes | Serving 8

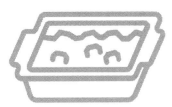

Ingredients:

♦ 1 bag Frozen Hash Brown Potatoes (907 g /32 oz)

♦ 1 lb (500 g) bacon, sausage or ham, diced & cooked

♦ 3 sliced onions

♦ 8 oz (225 g) cheddar cheese, grated

♦ ½ diced green bell pepper

♦ ½ diced red bell pepper

♦ 1 cup Milk

♦ 12 Eggs

♦ 1 tsp dry mustard

♦ salt and pepper to taste

Preparation:

1. Grease the slow cooker. Layer starting with half the hash browns, meat, onions, cheese and peppers. Repeat layers ending with cheese on top.

2. Whisk eggs, dry mustard, milk, salt & pepper and pour the mixture over the Ingredients: in the cooker

3. Cook on high for 2½ - 3 hours or low for 7-8 hours.

Cheesy Breakfast Potatoes

Time: 4 hours 15 minutes | Serving 8

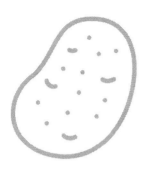

Ingredients:

♦ 3 peeled potatoes, diced

♦ 1 diced onion

♦ 1 diced red bell pepper,

♦ 1 diced green bell pepper,

♦ 13 oz (370 g) thinly sliced smoked andouille chicken sausage

♦ 1 ½ cups cheddar cheese, shredded

♦ ½ cup sour cream

♦ ¼ tsp dried basil

♦ ¼ tsp dried oregano

♦ 10 ¾ oz (305 g) can condense cream of chicken soup

♦ 2 tbsp parsley leaves, chopped

♦ Salt & ground black pepper

Preparation:

1. Add potatoes, bell peppers, onion, chicken sausage, sour cream, cheese, basil, oregano, and chicken soup in a cooker, with salt & pepper

2. Cover and cook on low for 4 to 5 hours or high for 2 to 3 hours.

3. Garnished with parsley to serve.

Breakfast Quinoa

Time: 8hrs 05 minutes | Serving 4

Ingredients:

♦ 1cup quinoa, uncooked

♦ 2 cups water

♦ 2 tbsp raw honey

♦ 1 cup canned coconut milk

♦ 1/4 tsp salt

♦ Milk, if desired

♦ Nuts, berries, fruit, honey, vanilla extract, cinnamon for toppings

Preparation:

1. Rinse quinoa under cold water

2. Add quinoa, water, coconut milk, honey and salt to cooker. Cover and cook on low for 8 hours. Serve hot with milk to taste and desired toppings.

Creamy Banana French Toast

Time: 4hrs 10 minutes | Serving 2

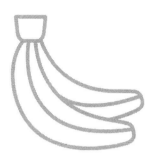

Ingredients:

- 1 slightly stale 1-inch (2 cm) slices of French baguette
- 4 oz (113 g) cream cheese
- 2 tbsp brown sugar
- 3 or 4 sliced bananas
- ½ cup walnuts or pecans, chopped

- 3 eggs
- ⅓ cup honey
- ¼ cup skim milk
- 1 tsp cinnamon
- pinch of nutmeg
- ½ tbsp pure vanilla extract
- 2 tbsp thin slices of butter

Preparation:

1. Lightly grease slow cooker with cooking spray
2. Spread bread on both sides with cream cheese and arrange in one layer on bottom of cooker
3. Cover bread with banana slice and sprinkle with brown sugar and nuts. Top with butter slices & set one side
4. Whisk eggs, add milk, honey, nutmeg, cinnamon, & vanilla extract. Mix well and pour over bread
5. Cook on low for 3-4 hours or high for up to 2½ hours. Remove lid and, if not serving immediately, set to warm. Serve drizzled with honey.

Apple Oatmeal

Time: 9hrs 20 minutes | Serving 8

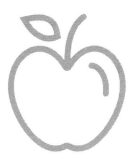

Ingredients:

♦ ¼ cup brown sugar

♦ 2 cups milk

♦ 2 tbsp honey

♦ 2 tbsp melted butter

♦ Pinch salt

♦ ½ tsp cinnamon

♦ 1 cup regular, non-instant oats

♦ 1 cup chopped apple

♦ ½ cup chopped dates, or raisins, or dried cranberries

♦ ½ cup chopped walnuts or pecans

Preparation:

1. Lightly grease a slow cooker with cooking spray

2. Mix milk, brown sugar, honey, melted butter, salt, and cinnamon in the slow cooker

3. Add oats, apple, dates or raisins or dried cranberries, and the walnuts or pecans and cover the slow cooker. Cook on low for 5 to 7 hours until oatmeal is cooked. Serve hot.

Sausage Breakfast Burritos

Time: 8hrs 25 minutes | Serving 10

Ingredients:

♦ 2 lbs (1 kg) uncooked breakfast sausage

♦ 1 package of frozen hash browns

♦ 14 eggs

♦ Salt & pepper

♦ 2 tbsp hot sauce

♦ 1 diced onion

♦ 1 diced pepper

♦ 1 cup shredded Mexican blend cheese

♦ 2 sliced avocados

♦ Salsa & sour cream for garnish

♦ 8 to 10 burrito-size tortillas

Preparation:

1. Lightly grease cooker with cooking spray. Layer frozen hash browns on bottom, sprinkled with green pepper and onions

2. Cook the breakfast sausage in pan until brown. Do not to overcook as it will cook further in the slow cooker. Drain the excess oil

3. Beat the eggs with cheese, hot sauce, pepper, and season salt and pour over the onions and hash browns. Top with cooked breakfast sausage

4. Cook on low for 8 hours overnight. Make sure all Ingredients: are completely combined

5. Warm the tortillas, to serve place the sliced avocado, shredded cheese, sour cream, and salsa into bowls.

Cobbler

Time: 6hrs 15 minutes | Serving 4

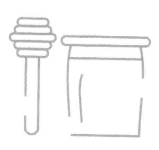

Ingredients:

♦ 2 cups granola cereal

♦ 3 cups tart apples, peeled and sliced

♦ 1 tsp cinnamon

♦ ¼ cup honey

♦ 3 tbsp butter, melted

Preparation:

1. Lightly grease a slow cooker with cooking spray

2. Place apples in slow cooker, sprinkled with cinnamon and granola. Stir honey and butter together and drizzle it over the apple mixture. Mix everything together

3. Cover and cook on low for 5 to 7 hours, until tender

4. Serve as preferred, with fruit yogurt or ice cream.

Yogurt

Time: 4hrs 30 minutes | Serving 6

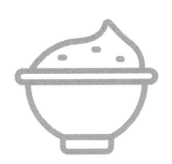

Ingredients:

♦ ½ Gallon (1.8 L) Whole Organic Milk
♦ ½ Cup Plain Yogurt

Preparation:

1. Add ½ gallon milk into a slow cooker. Insert a cooking thermometer into a slow cooker and click "boil". Stir the milk to avoid burning. When the temperature reaches 200°F (93°C), turn the cooker off

2. Remove one cup of the milk and mix in bowl with ½ cup plain yogurt. Once milk cools to 112°F (45°C), return to cooker. Whisk well

3. Cover and set aside for 4 hours. Then pour yoghurt in jars and refrigerate. As it chills, it will set.

Denver Omelette Breakfast Pie

Time: 3 hours | Serving 8

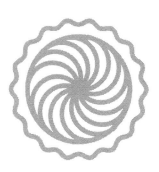

Ingredients:

- 8 oz (225 g) refrigerated crescent dough sheet
- ½ cup green bell pepper, chopped
- ½ cup onion, chopped
- ¾ cup ham, chopped
- 1 cup mushrooms, sliced
- 4 oz (110 g) grated Cheddar cheese
- 6 eggs
- Salt and red pepper flakes
- Chopped chives

Preparation:

1. Lightly grease slow cooker with cooking spray and evenly line with crescent dough, 1" (2 ½ cm) up the sides

2. Mix mushrooms, onion, ham, bell pepper, and ½ cup cheese. Spread half the mixture on crescent dough

3. Beat eggs, salt and pepper flakes together well. Add mixture on ham and vegetable mixture, carefully, keeping egg within crescent-lined bottom. Top with remaining ham, vegetables, and beaten eggs. Press mixture into eggs with a spatula. Add remining ½ cup cheese.

4. Cover cooker first with kitchen towel folded in half and then lid. Cook on low for 1 ½ hours. Keeping it covered, rotate inside of cooker 180˚. Cook for 1 to 1½ hrs, until eggs are set and dough golden. Let stand for 10 minutes and then cut.

5. Slice to serve and garnish with chives.

Hot Chocolate Oatmeal

Time: 6hrs 10 minutes| Serving 6

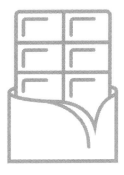

Ingredients:

♦ 5 cups water

♦ 1 cup oats

♦ ⅓ cup instant cocoa mix

♦ ⅓ cup packed brown sugar

♦ ½ teaspoon salt

♦ Chocolate chips and additional brown sugar

Preparation:

1. Lightly grease slow cooker with cooking spray

2. Mix water and oats and pour into cooker. Cover; cook on low for 6 hours, until cooked through

3. Stir in ⅓ cup brown sugar, instant cocoa mix and salt before serving. Serve with chocolate chips and additional brown sugar.

MAIN MEAL RECIPES

Easy Balsamic Beef

Time: 7hrs 5 minutes| Serving 8

Ingredients:

♦ 2-3 lb (1-1 ½ kg) beef chuck or roast
♦ 1 cup low sodium beef broth
♦ 1 tbsp Worcestershire sauce
♦ ⅓ cup balsamic vinegar
♦ ¼ cup light brown sugar
♦ 1 tbsp soy sauce
♦ 3-4 garlic cloves, minced
♦ Salt and pepper

Preparation:

1. Mix together broth, balsamic vinegar, Worcestershire sauce, brown sugar, soy sauce, garlic, salt, and pepper

2. Place roast in cooker with broth mixture. Cover and cook on low for 6 to 8 hours or high for 4 hours. Shred meat when done, remove from cooker and set one side

3. Simmer liquid from cooker in pan for 5-10 minutes to thicken. Drizzle over meat and serve immediately.

Korean Beef

Time: 8hrs 40 minutes| Serving 8

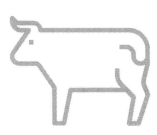

Ingredients:

- 1 cup beef broth
- ½ cup soy sauce
- ½ cup brown sugar
- 1 tbsp sesame oil
- 4 garlic cloves, grated
- 1 tbsp ginger, grated
- 1 tbsp rice wine vinegar
- 1 tsp Sriracha, or more
- ½ tsp white pepper
- ½ tsp onion powder
- 3lb (1 ½ kg)boneless beef chuck roast, in 1" (2½ cm) cubes
- 2 tbsp corn-starch
- 2 thinly sliced onions
- 1 tsp sesame seeds

Preparation:

1. Whisk beef broth, soy sauce, garlic, sugar, sesame oil, rice wine vinegar, ginger, Sriracha, onion powder and pepper together

2. Place chuck roast in cooker, stir in beef broth mixture until well mixed. Cover and cook on high for 3 to 4 hours or on low for 7 to 8hours

3. Whisk together corn-starch and ¼ cup water. Add to cooker, cover and cook on high for 30 minutes, until sauce has thickened

4. Serve immediately, garnished with sesame seeds and onions, if desired.

Beef Vegetable Stew

Time: 6hrs 50 minutes| Serving 8

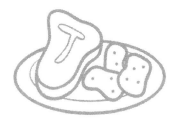

Ingredients:

- 1½ lb (700 g) boneless beef chuck roast, 1-inch (2 ½ cm) cubes
- 3 peeled potatoes, cubed
- 3 cups water
- 1 ½ cups baby carrots
- 10 ¾ oz (4.8 kg) undiluted condensed tomato soup
- 1 chopped celery rib
- 1 chopped onion
- 2 tbsp Worcestershire sauce
- 2 tsp beef bouillon granules
- 1 tbsp browning sauce (optional)
- 1 garlic clove, minced
- 1 tsp sugar
- Salt and pepper
- ¼ cup corn-starch
- 2 cups thawed frozen peas
- ¾cup cold water

Preparation:

1. Add the beef, potatoes, water, carrots, soup, onion, celery, Worcester-shire sauce, browning sauce (optional), bouillon granules, sugar, garlic, salt and pepper to cooker. Cover and cook on low for 6 to 8 hours

2. Mix corn-starch and cold water until smooth, stir into stew. Cover and cook until thickened on high for 30 minutes. Add peas and heat through

3. Serve hot.

Spaghetti and Meatballs

Time: 6 hrs | Serving 6

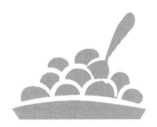

Ingredients:

♦ 2 tbsp grated Parmesan and Romano cheese blend

♦ 1 cup bread crumbs

♦ 2 eggs

♦ 2 lbs (1 kg) ground beef

♦ Salt and pepper

♦ SAUCE:

♦ 1 finely chopped green pepper

♦ 1 finely chopped onion

♦ 2 cans (14 ½ oz/410 g each) tomatoes, diced & undrained

♦ 3 x 15 oz(425g) cans tomato sauce

♦ 1 can (6 oz/170 g) tomato paste

♦ 6minced garlic cloves

♦ 2 bay leaves

♦ 1 tsp dried basil, oregano and parsley flakes

♦ Salt and pepper and red pepper flakes Hot cooked spaghetti

Preparation:

1. Mix bread crumbs, cheese, pepper and salt, followed by beaten eggs. Shape beef into 1½" (4 cm) balls and cook in pan until browned. Drain

2. Place the bread crumb mixture in cooker, stir in garlic and seasonings. Add meatballs, gently coating them. Cover and cook on low for to 6 hours, until cooked through

3. Before serving with spaghetti, remove bay leaves.

Honey, Lime & Ginger Pork

Time: 8 hrs 10 minutes| Serving 8

Ingredients:

- 2½ lbs (1 kg) pork loin
- 1 tbsp Olive oil
- Salt and Pepper
- Marinade:
- ¼ cup soy sauce
- ½ cup honey
- 1 tbsp Worcestershire Sauce
- ½ tsp ground ginger or 1 tbsp fresh ginger
- 2 garlic cloves, minced
- 1 juiced lime
- 2 tbsp corn-starch
- Fresh lime wedges & chopped cilantro (optional)

Preparation:

1. Season pork and sear it in oil heated over medium heat, until outside edge blackens. Put pork in bottom of cooker

2. Whisk honey, Worcestershire sauce, soy sauce, lime juice, garlic cloves, and ginger together and pour it over pork. Cook on low for 6 to 8 hours, or on high for 4 to 6 hours

3. Remove and pour juices into saucepan. Cook marinade over medium-high heat. Whisk in corn-starch and cook to thicken. Pour over the pork and garnish as preferred.

Texan Style Pulled Pork

Time: 5 hrs 15 minutes| Serving 8

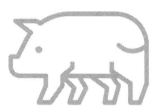

Ingredients:

- 4 lbs (1.8 kg) pork shoulder roast
- 1 tsp vegetable oil
- 1 cup barbeque sauce
- ½ cup chicken broth
- ½ cup apple cider vinegar
- ¼ cup light brown sugar
- 1 tbsp prepared yellow mustard
- 1 tbsp chili powder
- 1 tbsp Worcestershire sauce
- 1 large chopped onion
- 1 ½ tsp dried thyme
- 2 crushed garlic cloves
- 8 hamburger rolls, halved
- 2 tbsp butter

Preparation:

1. Pour vegetable oil in cooker and add pork roast, apple cider vinegar, barbecue sauce, and chicken broth. Stir in sugar, Worcestershire sauce, mustard, chili powder, onion, and garlic, thyme

2. Cover and cook for 5 to 6 hours on high until it shreds easily. Remove meat from cooker, shred using two forks. Replace shredded pork in a cooker. Stir meat into juices

3. Butter hamburger rolls and toast them butter side down over medium heat until golden. Fill rolls with pork.

Pork Roast

Time: 6 hrs 9 minutes| Serving 8

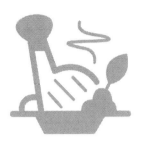

Ingredients:

♦ 3-4 lb (1.3-1.8 kg) pork roast
♦ 1 cup broth
♦ ¼ cup of soy sauce
♦ ¼ cup balsamic vinegar
♦ 2 tsp corn-starch
♦ 2 tbsp honey
♦ 2 tsp minced garlic

Preparation:

1. Place roast in a slow cooker. Mix all Ingredients: but corn-starch and pour over roast. Cook on low for 10 to 12 hours or on high for 6-8 hours, until in falls apart

2. Before serving, scoop about ¼ cup of the juice and strain into measuring cup

3. Whisk in the corn-starch and add juice to make up 1 cup. Microwave on high for 30 seconds, whisk again and drizzle over meat before serving.

Chipotle Pork Chops

Time: 4 hrs 15 minutes| Serving 8

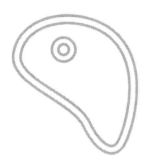

Ingredients:

- 8 pork loin chops, bone-in (7 oz/200 g each)
- 1 onion finely chopped
- ⅓ cup chipotle peppers, chopped, in adobo sauce
- ¼ cup brown sugar
- 2 minced garlic cloves
- 2 tbsp red wine vinegar
- Salt and pepper
- 1 15 oz can (425 g)tomato sauce
- 1 14 ½ oz can (410 g) undrained fire-roasted diced tomatoes

Toppings:

- 1 can (6 oz/170 g) french-fried onions
- ¼ cup fresh cilantro, mince

Preparation:

1. Add all Ingredients: but toppings to slow cooker. Cover and cook for 4-5 hours on low

2. Garnish with french-fried onions and cilantro to serve.

Brown Sugar and Garlic Chicken

Time: 4 hrs 5 minutes| Serving 5

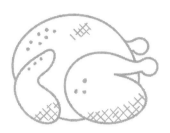

Ingredients:

- ♦ 5 chicken thighs
- ♦ 2 tbsp garlic, minced
- ♦ Salt and pepper
- ♦ ⅓ cup brown sugar

Preparation:

1. Cover chicken in salt, pepper, and garlic inside the cooker, and turn chicken skin side up

2. Sprinkle with brown sugar and cook on low for 8 hours or high for 4 hours.

Chicken Casserole

Time: 4 hrs 15 minutes| Serving 4

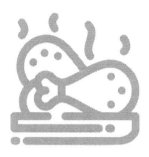

Ingredients:

- ♦ 1 tbsp butter
- ♦ 1 ½ tbsp flour
- ♦ ½ tbsp olive oil
- ♦ 1 finely chopped onion
- ♦ 23 oz (650 g) boneless and skinless chicken thigh fillets,
- ♦ 3 garlic cloves, crushed
- ♦ 14 oz (400 g) halved baby potatoes
- ♦ 2 diced sticks celery
- ♦ 2 diced carrots
- ♦ 2 chicken stock cubes in17 fl oz (500 ml) water
- ♦ 9 oz (250 g) quartered mushrooms
- ♦ ½ oz (15 g) dried porcini mushroom, soaked in 50ml boiling water
- ♦ 2 bay leaves
- ♦ 2 tsp Dijon mustard

Preparation:

1. Heat butter and olive oil in frying pan to cook onion until softened and almost caramelised, 8 to 10 minutes

2. Meanwhile combine flour, salt and pepper and toss chicken thighs in it. Cook garlic and chicken in pan for 4 to 5 mins

3. Place chicken, baby potatoes, celery sticks, chicken stock, carrots, mushrooms, porcini mushrooms, Dijon mustard and bay leaves in cooker

4. Stir well. Cook for 7 hours on low or on high for 4 hours

5. Remove bay leaves to serve with Dijon mustard on side.

Chicken Cacciatore

Time: 6 hours 10 minutes| Serving 6

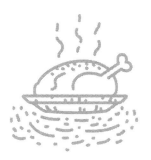

Ingredients:

♦ 2 lb (1 kg) chicken thighs, skin-on and bone-in
♦ Salt and pepper
♦ 2 chopped bell peppers
♦ 8 oz (225 g) sliced baby Bella mushrooms
♦ 2 garlic cloves, minced
♦ ½ cup chicken broth
♦ 1 28 oz can (790g) crushed tomatoes
♦ 1 tsp dried oregano
♦ ¼ tsp red pepper flakes
♦ ⅓ cup capers
♦ Cooked linguine

Preparation:

1. Placed well-seasoned chicken in a slow cooker, add peppers, mushrooms, garlic, tomatoes, and broth, and season with red pepper flakes, oregano, salt, and pepper

2. Cover and cook for 6 to 8 hours on low or on high for 3 to 4 hours

3. Remove chicken, add capers, stir and serve over cooked pasta.

Rotisserie Chicken

Time: 3 hours 15 minutes| Serving 4 - 6

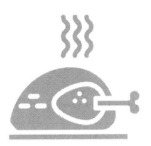

Ingredients:

♦ Cooking spray

♦ 2 tbsp brown sugar

♦ 1 tsp fresh thyme

♦ 1 tsp smoked paprika

♦ 1 ½ tsp chili powder

♦ 1 whole chicken, washed and seasoned with Salt and pepper

Preparation:

1. Lightly grease a slow cooker with cooking spray. Create a rack for the chicken by placing small rolled balls of aluminium foil in slow cooker

2. Whisk sugar, chili powder, paprika, and thyme together

3. Rub sugar mixture over chicken and place breast side up in slow cooker

4. Cook for 2½ to 3½ hours on high, until juices run clear

5. Remove chicken and crisp under oven grill for 3 or 4 minutes, until golden. Let stand for 10 minutes before slicing and serving.

SEAFOOD AND FISH RECIPES

Tuna Casserole

Time:4 hours 15 minutes| Serving 4 - 6

Ingredients:

♦ ⅓ cup chicken broth

♦ 2 cans cream of celery soup

♦ ⅔ cup milk

♦ 2 tbsp dried parsley flakes

♦ 1 package (10 ounces) thawed frozen peas

♦ 2x 7 oz cans (200 g) tuna (drained)

♦ 10 oz (285g) pasta, cooked

♦ 3 tbsp buttered breadcrumbs or potato chip crumbs

Preparation:

1. Lightly grease a slow cooker with cooking spray, bottom and sides

2. Mix soup, chicken broth, milk, parsley, vegetables, and tuna in a bowl. Pour mixture into prepared cooker with cooked pasta. Top with buttered breadcrumbs or potato chip crumb and cover

3. Cook for 4 to 6 hours on low. Serve hot.

Shrimp Boil

Time: up to 5 hours 15 minutes| Serving 4 - 6

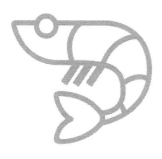

Ingredients:

♦ 1 ½ lbs (700 g) small potatoes, quartered

♦ 1 lb (500 g) kielbasa sausage, 1" (2 ½ cm) pieces

♦ 3 corn ears, cut into thirds

♦ ¼ cup Old Bay seasoning

♦ 6 cups water

♦ 6 garlic cloves, smashed

♦ 2 lbs (1 kg) raw shrimp, with tails, cleaned

For serving:

♦ Chopped parsley leaves

♦ Ground black pepper

♦ Melted butter

♦ Hot sauce

♦ 1 halved lemon, and wedges to serve

Preparation:

1. Layer potatoes on bottom of slow cooker in a single layer, adding sausage, corn, garlic and Old Bay seasoning

2. Squeeze lemon into cooker as well as squeezed halves. Add water to integrate Old Bay throughout. Do not stir

3. Cover and cook for 4-5 hours on high

4. Add shrimp and stir gently until just submerged. Cook for 10 to 15 minutes until opaque

5. Strain and serve. Add corn and top with parsley, Old Bay, and pepper. Serve with lemon wedges, melted butter, hot sauce, and cooking liquid for dipping.

Coconut Fish Curry

Time: up to 3 hours 5 minutes| Serving 4

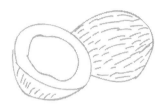

Ingredients:

- 2 garlic cloves finely chopped
- 1" (3 cm) peeled finely chopped ginger
- 1 seedless finely chopped red chilli
- 1 ½ tsp turmeric
- 1 stick lemongrass (squished)
- 13 ½ fl oz (400 ml) coconut milk
- 3 ½ oz (100 g) sliced mange tout
- 10½ oz (300 g) skinless, boneless cod loin, in 1" (2 cm) cubes
- 5 oz (150 g) broccoli florets
- To serve:
- Coriander
- Sliced red chilli

Preparation:

1. Toss ginger, garlic, red chilli, turmeric, coconut milk and lemongrass in cooker, as well as cod, mange tout and broccoli
2. Cook for 2-3 hours on low until cooked through
3. To serve, top with coriander and sliced chilli.

Shrimp Scampi

Time: up to 3 hours 5 minutes| Serving 4

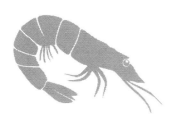

Ingredients:

♦ 2 lbs (1 kg) peeled shrimp
♦ ½ cup chicken broth
♦ ¾cup white wine
♦ ¼ cup shallots, minced
♦ 4 garlic cloves
♦ 3 tbsp olive oil
♦ ¼ tsp red pepper flakes
♦ 3 tbsp parsley
♦ 2 tbsp lemon juice
♦ Salt and pepper
♦ butter

Preparation:

1. Cook shrimp in butter for 2-3 minutes, making sure to keep stirring to sauté all sides of shrimp, and then refrigerate

2. Mix chicken broth, olive oil, white wine, garlic and shallots, and toss in slow cooker with red pepper flakes, parsley and lemon juice

3. Cover and cook for 2-3 hours on low

4. Add the refrigerated, cooked shrimp and sauce, cover and cook for 15 minutes longer.

Scalloped Potatoes with Salmon

Time: 9 hours 15 minutes| Serving 6

Ingredients:

♦ 4-5 peeled and sliced potatoes
♦ 3 tbsp flour
♦ Salt and pepper
♦ 1 16 oz can (450 g) salmon, flaked
♦ ½cup onion, chopped
♦ 1 x 10¾ oz an (305 g) cream of mushroom/cream of celery soup
♦ Dash of nutmeg
♦ ¼ cup water

Preparation:

1. Place half of the potatoes in greased the slow cooker. Sprinkle half of the flour over the potatoes, then sprinkle lightly with salt and pepper. Add half the flaked salmon, followed by half the onion. Repeat the layers

2. Mix soup and water. Pour mixture over potato and salmon. Sprinkle with just a dash of nutmeg

3. Cover and cook for 7-9 hours on low.

Sweet and Sour Shrimp

Time: 5 hours 30 minutes| Serving 3 - 4

Ingredients:

- ♦ 1 pack of (6 oz/170 g) Chinese pea pods - frozen
- ♦ 1 x 14 oz can (400 g) pineapple chunks
- ♦ 1 cup chicken stock
- ♦ 2 tbsp corn starch
- ♦ 3 tbsp sugar
- ♦ ½ cup pineapple juice
- ♦ ½ tsp ground ginger
- ♦ 1 tbsp soy sauce
- ♦ 1 bag (16 oz/450 g) cooked shrimp, frozen
- ♦ 1 cup rice, cooked2 tbsp cider vinegar

Preparation:

1. Clean and drain pea pods in cold water until thawed. Drain pineapple and reserve ½ cup juice

2. Put pea pods and pineapple in slow cooker

3. Mix corn-starch, sugar, chicken stock, soy sauce, ½ cup pineapple juice, and ginger together and bring to boil for a minute, stirring constantly until thickened

4. Stir sauce gently over pea pods and pineapple. Cover and cook for 3-4 hours on low, add shrimp and cook for 15 to 20 minutes, until hot. Add vinegar and stir

5. Serve hot with cooked rice.

Salmon

Time: up to 2 hours 15 minutes| Serving 3 - 6

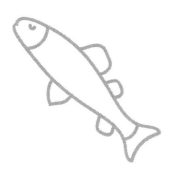

Ingredients:

♦ 1-2 lbs (½ kg-1 kg) salmon fillets, skin-on
♦ Salt and black pepper
♦ Spice
♦ Sliced lemon
♦ Sliced vegetables (e.g.: fennel, onions, celery
♦ 1 cup of either broth, water, wine, cider, beer, or a mixture

Preparation:

1. Line slow cooker interior with aluminium foil to lift salmon out easier
2. Cut salmon into individual-serving size and season the flesh as desired, rubbing in with fingers
3. Layer bottom of cooker with lemon and sliced aromatics before placing the larger salmon piece, skin-side down, on top, topping with more lemon slices and aromatics
4. Pour liquid over salmon, enough to barely cover
5. Cover and cook on low for 1-2 hours. Check after 1 hour and every 20 minutes thereafter until done. To remove, lift salmon by the aluminium foil, tilting slightly to drain liquid
6. Serve immediately

Chicken and Shrimp with Fettuccine

Time: 5 hours 15 minutes| Serving 6

Ingredients:

♦ 1 lb (500g) chicken breasts, boneless chunks
♦ 1lb (½ kg) chicken thighs, boneless chunks
♦ 1 cup onion, chopped
♦ 2 tbsp extra virgin olive oil
♦ 2 garlic cloves, minced
♦ ¼ cup parsley, minced
♦ 1 can (15 oz/425 g) tomato sauce
♦ ½ cup white wine
♦ 1 tsp dried basil
♦ 1lb (½ kg) shrimp, peeled and deveined
♦ salt and black pepper
♦ 1 lb (500g) pasta

Preparation:

1. Cook chicken chunks until lightly browned in olive oil heated over medium heat. Move to slow cooker

2. Add more oil to pan to sauté onion, garlic, and parsley for a minute. Remove from heat, stir in wine, tomato sauce, and basil, and pour over chicken. Cover and cook on low for 4-5 hours

3. Add shrimp to cooker, cover and cook on low for 1 hour. Season to taste

4. Serve with cooked pasta.

Shrimp Chowder

Time: 6 hours 15 minutes| Serving 6

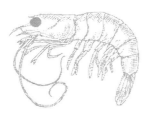

Ingredients:

♦ 2 lbs (1 kg) frozen fish, thawed

♦ ¼ lb (110 g) bacon

♦ 1 chopped onion

♦ 4 peeled and cubed red-skinned potatoes

♦ 2 cups water

♦ Salt and black pepper

♦ 1 can (12 oz/340 g) evaporated milk

Preparation:

1. Place bite sized pieces of thawed fish fillets in slow cooker

2. Dice bacon/salt pork and fry in heavy-based pan with chopped onion until the meat is cooked and onion is golden. Drain off excess fat and add bacon and onion mixture to fish

3. Add potatoes, water, salt, and pepper, cover and cook for 5 to 6 hours on low, until tender. Add evaporated milk and cook for 30 minutes to 1 hour

4. Serve hot.

VEGETABLES

Vegetables

Time: 7 hours 10 minutes| Serving 8

Ingredients:

♦ 4 celery ribs, 1" (2½ cm)

♦ 4 small carrots, 1" (2½ cm)

♦ 2 tomatoes, in chunks

♦ 2 thinly sliced onions

♦ 2 cups green beans, 1" (2½ cm)

♦ 1 green pepper, 1" (2½ cm)

♦ ¼ cup melted butter

♦ 1 tbsp sugar

♦ 3 tbsp quick-cooking tapioca

♦ Salt and pepper

Preparation:

1. Toss all vegetables in slow cooker

2. Mix butter, sugar, tapioca, salt and pepper and pour over vegetables, stirring well

3. Cover and cook on low for 7-8 hours.

Chicken and Broccoli

Time: 5 hours 30 minutes| Serving 4

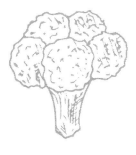

Ingredients:

♦ 2 garlic cloves, minced

♦ 1 tsp ginger, minced

♦ ¼ cup soy sauce

♦ ¼ cup honey

♦ ¼cup water

♦ 1 tbsp ketchup

♦ 2 tbsp rice wine vinegar

♦ 1 tsp sesame oil

♦ 1 tbsp Sriracha

♦ 2 lbs (1 kg) chicken breasts, boneless and skinless

♦ Salt and black pepper

♦ 1 head broccoli, cut into florets

♦ 1 tbsp corn starch

♦ For garnish:

♦ Thinly sliced green onions

♦ Toasted sesame seeds

♦ Cooked brown rice, for serving

Preparation:

1. Mix ginger, garlic, soy sauce, vinegar, honey, ketchup, Sriracha, and sesame oil together

2. Season chicken and toss in slow cooker with the sauce, combining well. Cook for 4 hours on low, until cooked through

3. Mix corn-starch and water and stir into cooker to thicken sauce. Add broccoli and cook for 1 hour

4. Put chicken on cutting board and cut into small pieces before returning to slow cooker, tossing to mix

5. Serve chicken and broccoli on cooked rice, garnished with onions and sesame seeds

Quinoa and vegetables

Time: 4 hours 10 minutes| Serving 4

Ingredients:

- 1½ cups Quinoa
- 3 cups Chicken/Vegetable Stock
- 1 tbsp olive oil
- 1 chopped onion
- 1 chopped carrot
- 1 chopped sweet red pepper
- 1 cup green beans, chopped
- 2 minced garlic cloves
- ¼ tsp pepper
- 1 tsp cilantro
- Garlic, salt, seasoned salt, or any spice of your choice

Preparation:

1. Put rinsed quinoa coated in olive oil into slow cooker, and stir in broth, veggies, pepper and garlic. Keep cilantro for serving

2. Cover and cook for 4-6 hours on low, or for 2-4 hours on high. There should be no liquid left in the Quinoa and you should be able to fluff it with a fork

3. Top with fresh cilantro and serve.

Vegetable & Chickpea Curry

Time: 8 hours 10 min| Serving 4

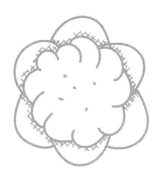

Ingredients:

- 2 cups quartered Brussels sprouts
- 4 cups cauliflower, cut in florets
- 1 diced red pepper
- 1 peeled and diced sweet potato
- 1 diced onion
- 15 oz can (425 g) chickpeas, drained
- 15 oz can (425 g) tomato sauce
- ½ cup chicken/ vegetable broth
- ½ cup light coconut milk
- 1 tbsp cumin
- 1 tbsp turmeric
- 1 tbsp curry powder
- ½ cup frozen green peas
- ½ tsp cayenne optional
- salt and pepper
- Garnishing (optional):
- Plain yogurt cilantro, scallions and sriracha

Preparation:

1. Cook veg, tomato sauce, coconut milk, chickpeas, chicken broth and spices in slow cooker for 8 hours on low or on high for 4 hours
2. Stir in green peas to warm and season accordingly
3. Serve with brown rice, yogurt, scallions and cilantro.

SOUPS, STEWS & CHILIS

Fisherman's Stew (Cioppino)

Time: 8 hours 20 mins| Serving 6

Ingredients:

- 1 can (28 oz/790 g) crushed tomatoes, juice incl.
- 1 cup dry white wine
- 1 can (8 oz/225 g) tomato sauce
- ½ cup chopped onion
- ½ cup chopped parsley
- ⅓ cup olive oil
- 3 garlic cloves minced
- 1 chopped hot pepper,
- 1 chopped green pepper
- 1 tsp thyme
- Salt and pepper
- 1 tsp oregano
- 2 tsp basil
- ½ tsp paprika
- ½ tsp cayenne pepper
- For Seafood:
- 1 fillet of white fish, cubed
- 1 dozen prawns
- 1 dozen scallops
- 1 dozen mussels
- 1 dozen clams
- 1 cup crab meat, if desired

Preparation:

1. Place all Ingredients: but seafood in a slow cooker
2. Gently stir, cover, and cook on low for 6 to 8 hours. Add seafood 30 minutes before serving
3. Turn heat to high and gently stir occasionally, avoid tearing apart the fish pieces
4. Serve hot and enjoy!

Chicken Tortilla Soup

Time: 5 hours 15 minutes| Serving 6

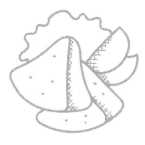

Ingredients:

- ♦ 1 can (15 oz/425 g) black beans, rinsed
- ♦ 1 lb (500 g) chicken breasts, skinless, boneless
- ♦ 2 chopped bell peppers
- ♦ 1 cup frozen corn
- ♦ 1 chopped onion
- ♦ 1 can (15 oz/425 g) fire-roasted tomatoes
- ♦ ¼ cup chopped coriander, and extra for garnish
- ♦ 3 minced garlic cloves
- ♦ 1 tbsp chili powder
- ♦ 1 tbsp cumin
- ♦ Salt
- ♦ 1 cup shredded cheese
- ♦ 2 cups chicken broth
- ♦ 1 tbsp extra-virgin olive oil
- ♦ 3 small corn tortillas
- ♦ For serving:
- ♦ Sliced avocado
- ♦ Sour cream
- ♦ Lime wedges

Preparation:

1. Combine chicken, black beans, corn, peppers, onion, fire-roasted tomatoes, cilantro, garlic, cumin, chili powder, salt, and chicken broth into the slow cooker

2. Cover and cook for 5-6 hours on low, until chicken is falling apart

3. Shred chicken with a fork. Sprinkle cheese over top and cover for 5 minutes, to melt

4. Meanwhile cook tortilla strips in hot oil for 3 minutes, until crispy and golden in a heavy-based pan, over medium heat. Remove onto paper towel-lined and season with salt

5. Serve soup with tortilla crisps, sour cream, avocado, coriander, and lime.

Chicken Noodle Soup

Time: 6 hours 40 minutes| Serving 6 - 8

Ingredients:

- 1 ½ lb (700 g) chicken breasts, boneless and skinless
- 1 chopped onion
- 3 peeled and cut carrots
- 2 sliced celery stalks
- 4 sprigs fresh thyme
- 4 sprigs fresh rosemary
- 1 bay leaf
- 3 minced garlic cloves
- 10 cups chicken broth
- Salt and black pepper
- 8 oz (225 g) egg noodles

Preparation:

1. Mix chicken, carrots, celery, onion, rosemary, thyme, garlic, salt and pepper and bay leaf in slow cooker and pour in broth

2. Cover and cook 6 to 8 hours on low. Remove chicken and shred with two forks. Discard bay leaf and herbs, return chicken to cooker and add noodles

3. Cook on low, 20 to 30 minutes, covered, until al dente.

Vegetable Soup

Time: 6 hours 40 minutes| Serving 8

Ingredients:

♦ 1 diced onion

♦ 2 tbsp olive oil

♦ 3 sliced celery ribs

♦ 4 sliced carrots

♦ 4 garlic cloves minced

♦ 3 cups potatoes, diced½ inch

♦ ¼ cup parsley, chopped

♦ 28 oz (800g) can diced tomatoes, undrained

♦ 2 tbsp tomato paste

♦ 2 cups chopped green beans, frozen or fresh

♦ 2 bay leaves

♦ ½ tsp dried thyme

♦ 1 tsp smoked paprika

♦ Salt and pepper

♦ ½ tsp dried oregano

♦ ½ tsp dried basil

♦ 8 cups vegetable broth

♦ 1 cup corn kernels, frozen/fresh

♦ To garnish: chopped dill/parsley

♦ To serve: Fresh lemon juice

Preparation:

1. Cook onions, celery and carrots for 4 minutes in heated olive oil over medium-high heat. After stirring in in garlic and fresh parsley, cook for 30 seconds more

2. Toss in slow cooker, and gently stir in diced tomatoes, potatoes, green beans, tomato paste, bay leaves, smoked paprika, salt, thyme, basil, oregano, pepper, and vegetable broth.

3. Cover and cook for 6 hours on low, or for 3 hours on high. Add corn during final 30 minutes

4. Ladle into serving bowls, garnished with fresh dill or parsley, plus a squeeze of fresh lemon juice and serve.

Beef Stew

Time: 4 hours 20 minutes| Serving 4

Ingredients:

- 30 oz (900 g) beef
- 2 finely chopped celery sticks
- 1 chopped onion
- 2 tbsp rapeseed oil
- 3 carrots, halved in chunks
- 2 bay leaves
- ½ pack thyme
- Pepper, to taste
- 2 tbsp Worcestershire sauce
- 2 tbsp tomato purée
- 20 fl oz (600ml) boiling water
- 2 tsp corn-flour (optional)
- 2 beef stock cubes
- ½ small bunch parsley, chopped
- Buttery mash, to serve

Preparation:

1. Fry the onion and celery in oil over a low heat until softened, for about 5 minutes. Add the carrots, bay and thyme, fry for 2 minutes, and stir in Worcestershire sauce and purée

2. Add boiling water, stir and move everything into a slow cooker. Break stock cubes in, stir, and season with pepper

3. Fry beef in frying pan in batches in leftover oil until well browned, then move into the slow cooker. Cook for 8-10 hours on low, or on high for 4 hours

4. To thicken the gravy, mix the corn flour with dash of cold water to make a paste. Stir in 2 tbsp of slow cooker liquid. Stir mixture into cooker, cook on high for 30 minutes, Stir in parsley and season again to taste.

5. Serve with mash, if desired.

Chili

Time: 6 hours 15 minutes| Serving 8

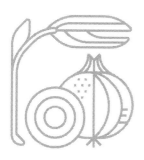

Ingredients:

- 2 lbs (1 kg) ground beef
- 1 chopped onion
- 2 tbsp tomato paste
- 1 28 oz can (800 g) crushed tomatoes
- 2x 15 oz cans (425 g) kidney beans, drained and rinsed
- 1 cup beer (or water)
- 4 minced garlic cloves
- 1 tsp dried oregano
- 1 tsp ground cumin
- 1 tbsp chili powder
- ½ tsp paprika
- Pinch cayenne pepper, if desired
- Kosher salt
- Ground black pepper
- Optional for Serving:
- Shredded cheddar
- Fritos
- Thinly sliced onions

Preparation:

1. Heat a heavy-based pan over medium-high heat, add beef and onion and cook for 4 minutes, until browned. Drain the fat and mix in tomato paste

2. Mix beef, onion, kidney beans, crushed tomatoes, beer, paprika, garlic, cumin, oregano, chili powder, and cayenne to cooker and season

3. Cook for 6-8 hours on low. Add seasonings as desired. Serve with cheese, Fritos, and green onions, if using.

Beef Chili

Time: 3 hours 15 minutes| Serving 8

Ingredients:

- ♦ 2 lbs (1 kg) lean ground beef
- ♦ 3 garlic cloves, minced
- ♦ 1 chopped onion
- ♦ 29 oz can (820 g) diced tomatoes, not drained
- ♦ 2 cans 16 oz (450 g) red kidney beans, drained
- ♦ ¼cup tomato paste
- ♦ 3 tbsp chili powder
- ♦ Salt and black pepper
- ♦ 1 tsp ground cumin
- ♦ 1 jalapeno, minced (if desired)
- ♦ ½ cup saltine cracker crumbs, finely ground

Preparation:

1. Cook beef and onion over medium-high heat until browned and add to slow cooker with remaining Ingredients:
2. Cook for 3 hours on high or on low heat for 6 hours.

DESSERTS & SNACKS

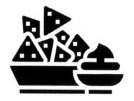

Appetiser Meatballs

Time: 3 hours 20 minutes| Makes 24

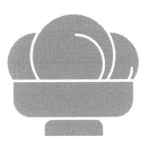

Ingredients:

♦ 4 dozen frozen meatballs

♦ 1 tbsp dried minced onion

♦ 1 cup currant jelly

♦ 1 ½ cups barbecue sauce

♦ If desired, ½ cup sliced onion, or chopped cilantro

Preparation:

1. Place frozen meatballs in slow cooker

2. Whisk onion, currant jelly, and barbecue sauce to blend thoroughly

3. Pour sauce mixture in cooker and mix to coat meatballs, cover and cook for 3-4 hours on low or high for 1 ½-2 hours

4. Serve hot in serving dish or directly from slow cooker. Garnish with sliced onion or chopped cilantro, if desired.

Broccoli Cheese Dip

Time: 2 hours 7 minutes| 12-15 Portions

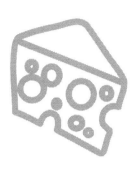

Ingredients:

♦ 1 ½ lbs (700 g) of fresh chopped broccoli, cooked

♦ 1 lb (500 g) plain Velveeta cheese, cubed

♦ 2 x 10oz cans (305 g) cream of mushroom soup

♦ ¼ cup sour cream

♦ ¾ tbsp garlic powder

Preparation:

1. Cook cheese cubes in slow cooker on low for 1 to 2 hours, until cheese melts

2. Mix the condensed soup, sour cream, garlic powder, chopped cooked broccoli, in a bowl

3. Stir soup and broccoli mixture into melted cheese and mix well

4. Once cooked, keep on low temp and serve with tortilla chips as dip.

Garlic and Ginger Chicken Wings

Time: 6 hours 15 minutes| Serving 4 - 6

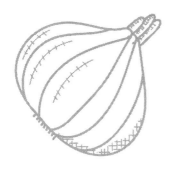

Ingredients:

♦ 12-18 whole chicken wings, washed, dried and with wing tips discarded
♦ 1 tsp ground ginger
♦ 2 minced garlic cloves
♦ ⅓ cup soy sauce
♦ 2 thinly sliced onions
♦ 2 tsp vegetable oil
♦ 1 tbsp honey
♦ If desired, top with thinly sliced onion, chopped cilantro or sesame seeds

Preparation:

1. Cut each wing in two at joint and toss into slow cooker
2. Mix garlic, soy sauce, ginger, sliced onions, honey, and vegetable oil and add to the slow cooker. Cover and cook on low for 6-8 hours
3. Top with chopped cilantro, sesame seeds, or diagonally sliced onion.

Brownie Pudding

Time: 2 hours 15 minutes| Serving 10

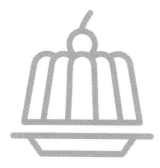

Ingredients:

♦ 1 box (15 oz/425 g) Brownie Mix

♦ 2 large eggs, water, and oil according to the brownie mix box

♦ ½ cup vegetable oil

♦ 3 tbsp water

♦ 1 box (3.4 oz/100 g) instant chocolate or chocolate fudge pudding mix

♦ 2 cups milk

♦ Ice cream or whipped cream for serving (if desired)

Preparation:

1. Lightly grease a slow cooker with cooking spray

2. Prepare brownie mix with eggs, oil, and water (as instructed on the box)and pour in prepared slow cooker

3. Mix pudding mix and milk until smooth. Pour carefully over the brownie mix in the slow cooker

4. Cover the slow cooker with paper towel and then the lid. Cook for 2-3 hours on high

5. Watch the edges; when they look slightly dry and done, the pudding is ready

6. Serve warm with whipped cream or ice cream.

Gingerbread Pudding Cake

Time: 2 hours 50 minutes| Serving 6

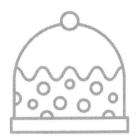

Ingredients:

- ¼ cup butter softened
- ¼ cup granulated sugar
- 1 egg
- 1 tsp vanilla
- ½ cup molasses
- 1 cup water
- ½ tsp ground cinnamon
- ¾ tsp baking soda
- ⅛ tsp nutmeg
- ½ tsp ground ginger
- Salt
- Topping:
- 6 tbsp brown sugar
- ¾ cup hot water
- ¼ cup melted butter
- 1¼ cups whole wheat flour

Preparation:

1. Beat butter and sugar with an electric mixer, until combined. Then add egg, beating until mixed. Add vanilla, molasses and water - beat to combine

2. Add flour, baking soda, cinnamon, ginger, salt and nutmeg and beat until well mixed. Pour into greased slow cooker

3. Sprinkle batter with brown sugar then combine hot water and melted butter and pour over brown sugar. Do not stir

4. Cover with the lid and cook for 2½ to 3 hours on high

5. Serve warm with ice cream or whipped cream.

KETO

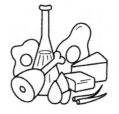

Chicken Tikka Masala

Time: 4 hours 30 minutes| Serving 4 - 6

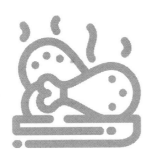

Ingredients:

♦ 2 lbs (1 kg) chicken thighs,
 boneless and skinless,
 in 1" (2 ½ cm) pieces

♦ ½cup plain yogurt (not Greek)

♦ 3 minced garlic cloves

♦ Salt

♦ 1 diced onion

♦ 1 tbsp ginger, peeled and minced

♦ 2 tsp garam masala

♦ 2 tsp ground coriander

♦ 1 tsp ground turmeric

♦ 1 tsp ground cumin

♦ 2 tbsp tomato paste

♦ ¾cup heavy cream or coconut milk

♦ 1 can (15 oz/425 g) drained diced tomatoes

♦ Chopped coriander

To serve:

♦ cooked rice or naan

Preparation:

1. Stir chicken, yogurt, and salt in slow cooker to combine

2. Simmer onion in frying pan, while stirring, for about 8 minutes until tender, in heated oil over medium heat

3. Add ginger, garlic, coriander, cumin, garam masala, and turmeric and cook for 1 minute, until aromatic. Add tomato paste and cook for 1 minute

4. Add drained tomatoes and salt and simmer. Move to slow cooker, stirring into chicken, cover and cook on low for 8 hours or high for 4 hours. Stir in cream/coconut milk. To thicken sauce, leave cooker uncovered and cook for 30 minutes on high

5. Season with salt to taste and serve garnished with coriander with rice/naan.

Carb-friendly Cabbage Roll Soup

Time: 3 hours 20 minutes| Serving 9

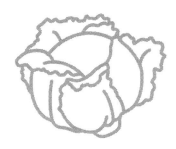

Ingredients:

♦ ½ cup chopped shallots
♦ 2 tbsp extra virgin olive oil
♦ 2 minced garlic cloves
♦ ½ cup chopped onion
♦ 2 lbs (1 kg) ground beef
♦ ½ tsp dried oregano
♦ 1 tsp dried parsley
♦ 1 tsp each salt and pepper
♦ 16 oz (450 g) low carb marinara sauce
♦ 5 cups beef broth8 cups sliced cabbage 2 cups riced cauliflower

Preparation:

1. Heat oil and garlic over medium-high heat, add onions and shallots, and cook until soft

2. Brown ground beef, add seasonings, marinara sauce and cauliflower rice, stir until coated

3. Pour beef into cooker, as well as the beef broth and cabbage. Stir to combine. Cook on low for 6 hours or high for 3 hours.

Pork Roast and Spicy Peanut Sauce

Time: up to 3 hours 15 minutes| Serving 6

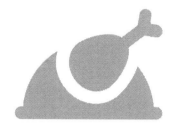

Ingredients:

- 2-3 lbs (1-1.3 kg) pork roast
- 2 tsp olive oil
- 1 tsp pork chop seasoning
- Sauce:
- 1 tbsp garlic, minced
- 1 tbsp ginger, minced
- ¼ cup smooth peanut butter
- 3 tbsp soy sauce
- 2 tsp chili garlic paste
- ¼ cup tomato sauce
- 3 tbsp sweetener
- ¼ cup chicken/vegetable stock

Preparation:

1. Remove visible fat from roast and cut into pieces and rub with pork chop seasoning. Brown well on all sides in oil heated in heavy frying pan over high heat. Place in slow cooker

2. Meanwhile add ginger, garlic, peanut butter, and tomato sauce and process until well mixed

3. Add soy sauce, sweetener, Chile garlic sauce, and stock. Process to mix

4. To add flavour (if desired),cook sauce in frying pan over low heat, scraping bits from base

5. Pour sauce over meat in cooker and cook on low for 2-3 hours, or until tender. Remove and let rest

6. Whisk to combine the sauce for 1 minute, if it has separated

7. Slice meat against the grain into ½" (1 ½ cm) thick slices and serve with drizzled sauce.

Keto Carnitas Lettuce Wraps

Time: up to 8 hrs 5 minutes| Serving 6

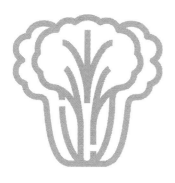

Ingredients:

♦ 3 ½ lbs (1 ½ kg) Pork Shoulder or Loin
♦ 4 minced garlic cloves
♦ 2 tbsp chili powder
♦ 4 tsp ground cumin
♦ 3 tsp dried oregano
♦ Salt and ground black pepper
♦ 2 chopped onions
♦ Juice from 2 oranges
♦ Juice from 2 limes
♦ Several heads of lettuce
♦ Fresh cilantro (if desired)
♦ Chopped red onion (if desired)
♦ Sour cream (if desired)

Preparation:

1. Mix chili powder, cumin, oregano, salt, and pepper and use to season the pork on all sides. Cook in slow cooker together with garlic, chopped onions, lime juice, and orange juice. Cover and cook for 8 hours on low or high for 4-5 hours

2. While in the slow cooker, shred meat using two forks

3. Serve on lettuce, garnished with cilantro, chopped red onion and sour cream.

Keto Crustless Pizza

Time: up to 4 hours 10 minutes| Serving 4

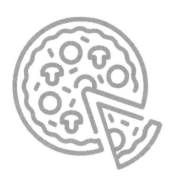

Ingredients:

♦ 2 lbs (1 kg) ground beef (browned)
♦ 2 cups mozzarella cheese
♦ 1 ½ cups pizza sauce
♦ 5-6 slices of mozzarella or provolone cheese
♦ Pizza toppings to taste

Preparation:

1. Lightly grease a slow cooker with cooking spray and add the browned ground beef and mozzarella. Stir to mix and spread evenly across the bottom

2. Top evenly with the pizza sauce in an even and add provolone cheese or extra mozzarella across the top

3. Top with selected pizza toppings. Cover and cook for 4 hours on low or high for 2 hours

4. Serve with parmesan cheese.

Mongolian Beef

Time: 35 minutes| Serving 6

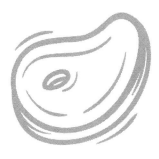

Ingredients:

♦ 2 lbs (1 kg)flank steak, sliced thinly against grain

♦ 3 garlic cloves, minced

♦ 2 tbsp avocado oil

♦ 2 tsp fresh ginger, grated or 1 tsp dried ginger

♦ ⅔ cup soy sauce/coconut aminos

♦ Pinch red pepper flakes, if desired

♦ ½ cup brown sugar

♦ 10-20 drops liquid stevia

♦ 1 tsp Xanthan Gum

♦ 2 thinly sliced onions (if desired)

♦ 2 tsp Sesame seeds, if desired)

Preparation:

1. Cook beef in heated oil in pan over high heat until outside is well seared

2. Move beef and cooking liquid to slow cooker. Add ginger, garlic, soy sauce, red pepper flakes, brown sugar, and 10 drops of liquid stevia

3. Cover and cook on low heat for 4-5 hours or high heat for 2-3 hours. Remove beef from cooker but leave liquid in slow cooker

4. Thicken liquid by stirring ¼ tsp xanthan gum in at a time, whisking after each addition. Stop adding at desired consistency

5. Return beef, stirring with sauce in the cooker. Serve topped with onions and sesame seeds.

LOW CARB DELIGHTS

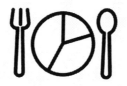

Creamy Chicken Marsala

Time: up to 4hours 50 minutes| Serving 4

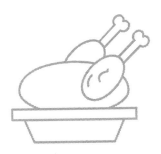

Ingredients:

♦ 4 (8 oz/225 g each) chicken breasts

♦ 8 oz (225 g) sliced cremini or button mushrooms

♦ 1 cup dry marsala wine

♦ salt and pepper

♦ ½ cup heavy whipping cream

Preparation:

1. Lightly grease slow cooker base with oil and add the chicken. Layer mushrooms and seasonings on top together with the wine

2. Cover and cook for 3-4 hours on high, until chicken is cooked. Remove from cooker and put one side

3. Stir in cream, whisking until thickened

4. Return chicken and mushrooms to cooker, cover and cook for 20-30 minutes.

Low Carb Beef Stroganoff

Time: 4hours 5 minutes| Serving 6

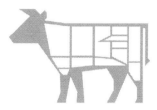

Ingredients:

- ♦ 1 onion, sliced and quartered
- ♦ 2 crushed garlic cloves
- ♦ 2 slices streaky bacon, diced
- ♦ 17 oz (500 g) beef stewing, cubed
- ♦ 1 tsp smoked paprika
- ♦ 3 tbsp tomato paste
- ♦ 8 ½ fl oz (250 ml) beef stock
- ♦ 9 oz (250 g) quartered mushrooms

Preparation:

1. Mix all Ingredients: in slow cooker together
2. Cook for 6-8 hours on low or high for 4-6 hours
3. Serve with sour cream (if desired).

Coq au Vin

Time: 5 hours 20 minutes| Serving 4

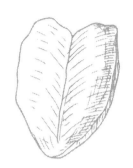

Ingredients:

- 4 (4 oz/110 g each) chicken breasts, boneless and skinless
- 3 chopped bacon strips
- ½ lb (250 g) sliced mushrooms
- 1 chopped onion
- 4 minced garlic cloves
- 1 bay leaf
- ⅓ cup all-purpose flour
- ½ cup red wine
- ½ cup chicken broth
- ½ tsp dried thyme
- ¼ tsp pepper
- Hot cooked noodles, optional

Preparation:

1. Crisp bacon over medium heat. And then remove using a slotted spoon. Drain on a paper towel. Brown both sides of chicken over medium heat in the drippings and then place into slow cooker

2. Cook mushrooms, garlic and onion in pan, stirring for 1 to 2 minutes until tender. Spoon over chicken, adding the bay leaf

3. Whisk the wine, broth, flour, thyme and pepper in a bowl until smooth and then pour over chicken

4. Cover and cook for 5 to 6 hours on low until chicken is tender, remove bay leaf and serve over oodles, if desired.

Carb-friendly Santa Fe Chicken

Time: 10 hours 10 minutes| Serving 8

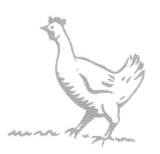

Ingredients:

- 1 can (14½ oz/420 g) chicken broth
- 1 can (15 oz/425 g) black beans, rinsed and drained
- 1 14 ½ oz can (420 g) diced tomatoes and green chili peppers
- 8oz (225 g) bag frozen corn
- 3 scallions, chopped
- ¼ cup chopped coriander,
- 1 tsp onion powder
- 1 tsp garlic powder
- 1 tsp cayenne pepper
- 1 tsp ground cumin
- Salt
- 1½ lbs (700 g) skinless and boneless chicken breast halves,

Preparation:

1. Add the black beans, chicken broth, diced tomatoes with green chile peppers, corn, cilantro, scallions, onion powder, garlic powder, cayenne pepper, cumin, and salt in slow cooker. Season chicken breast and place on top of bean mixture. Cook on low for 9 ½ hours

2. Move chicken from slow cooker to cutting board, shred, replace in slow cooker, and stir into the bean mixture. Continue cooking on low for a further 30 minutes

3. Serve hot.

Carb-friendly Beef Short Ribs

Time: 4 hours 15 minutes| Serving 12

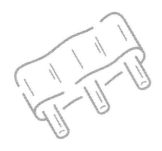

Ingredients:

♦ 4 lbs (1.8 kg) beef short ribs, cut to 2" (5 cm)
♦ 2 tbsp olive oil
♦ 1 cup beef broth
♦ 1 ½ cup chopped onion
♦ Salt and pepper
♦ 3 minced garlic cloves
♦ 2 tbsp tomato paste
♦ 2 tbsp Worcestershire sauce
♦ 1 ½ cup red wine
♦ Celery and carrots, if desired

Preparation:

1. Heat the oil in a pan over medium high heat. Season one side of ribs with salt and pepper and cook half the ribs, seasoned side down

2. Season top of ribs in pan, flip when browned, remove and leave one side while browning remaining meat cuts

3. Pour beef broth into slow cooker and add short ribs

4. Add remaining Ingredients: to same pan, bring to boil, cook for 5 minutes, pour over ribs in cooker, cover and cook on high for 4-6 hours or low for 8-10 hours.

Low Carb Butter Chicken

Time: 7 hours 15 minutes| Serving 4

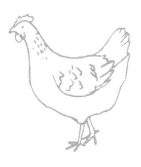

Ingredients:

♦ 2 tbsp Ghee

♦ 1 Onion, dices

♦ 3 minced garlic cloves

♦ 3 tbsp minced ginger

♦ 1 tbsp garam masala

♦ 6 tbsp tomato paste

♦ Salt

♦ 3 lbs (1.3 kg) chicken breast, in 2" (5 cm) pieces

♦ 1 tbsp lime juice

♦ Lime zest, if desired

♦ ½ cup chicken stock

♦ 1 cup coconut milk

♦ ⅛ cup cilantro and coriander leaves

Preparation:

1. Sauté onion, garlic, ginger and garam masala over medium-high heat in pan, add ghee, stir until spices are fragrant and onions are beginning to brown. Add tomato paste, cook until darkened and then sprinkle with salt

2. Mix together chicken pieces in slow cooker with lime zest (if desired), lime juice, chicken stock, coconut milk, onion and tomato paste mixture on low for 7 to 8 hours until chicken is tender

3. Serve with cauliflower rice, and top with cilantro.

VEGAN AND VEGETARIAN DISHES

Creamy chickpea & Veg Curry

Time: 3 hours 50 minutes| Serving 6

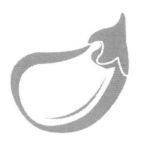

Ingredients:

- ♦ 2 tsp vegetable oil
- ♦ 1 cup vegetable liquid stock
- ♦ 2 tbsp curry paste
- ♦ 13 ½ fl oz can (400 ml) light coconut cream
- ♦ 1 red capsicum, in 1"(2cm) pieces
- ♦ 1 cauliflower, cut into florets
- ♦ 2 lbs (1 kg) pumpkin, in 2cm pieces
- ♦ 3 chopped tomatoes
- ♦ 1 grated Lebanese cucumber
- ♦ 10 ½ oz (300 g) halved green beans,
- ♦ 14 oz (400g) can chickpeas, drained, rinsed
- ♦ 2 tbsp fresh chopped coriander leaves
- ♦ Extra coriander for serving
- ♦ 1 cup Greek-style yoghurt
- ♦ 4 warmed naan breads

Preparation:

1. Stir curry paste in oil heated in medium pan over medium heat, stirring, for 30 seconds, until fragrant. Add stock, bring to boil, and simmer

2. Move to slow cooker, add coconut cream, pumpkin and capsicum, season, cover and cook for 1 hour 30 minutes on high or on low for 3 hours. Add cauliflower and tomato, cook for 15 minutes, and add beans and chickpeas. Cook for 30 minutes, until tender

3. Mix together cucumber, coriander and yoghurt in a bowl to serve with curry naan bread, and extra coriander.

Red Lentil Soup

Time: 4 hours 10 minutes| Serving 4

Ingredients:

- 2 tsp olive oil
- 2 diced carrots
- 1 diced onion
- 2 diced celery stalks
- 2 thinly sliced garlic cloves
- 1½" (4 cm) peeled, finely chopped ginger
- 3 tsp ground cumin
- 3 teaspoons ground coriander
- 1½ cups red lentils
- 34 fl oz (1 L) vegetable liquid stock
- 2 cups cold water
- For serving:
- Chopped coriander leaves
- Plain Greek-style yoghurt
- Warmed garlic naan bread

Preparation:

1. Cook onion, carrot and celery in heated oil in a large frying pan over medium heat for 5 minutes, stirring often . Cook for another minute after adding ginger and garlic

2. Add coriander and cumin and cook for 30 seconds while stirring. Move to slow cooker, and add lentils, stock, water, salt and pepper. Cover and cook for 4 hours on low

3. Serve with coriander and yoghurt, with naan bread.

Middle Eastern Chickpea Stew

Time: 6 hours 10 minutes| Serving 4

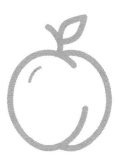

Ingredients:

- ½ cup dried chickpeas, rinsed, drained
- 14 oz (400 g) peeled orange sweet potato, cut into 1" (3 cm) pieces
- 1 finely chopped onion
- 1 thickly sliced carrot
- ½ cup dried apricots
- 8 fresh dates, pitted
- 2 cups vegetable liquid stock

- 14 oz (400 g) can diced tomatoes
- 3 tsp Moroccan seasoning paste
- 2 thickly sliced and halved (lengthways) zucchinis
- To serve:
- Cooked couscous
- Plain yoghurt
- Fresh coriander, if desired

Preparation:

1. Stir together chickpeas, sweet potato, onion, carrot, apricots, dates, stock, tomatoes and seasoning in slow cooker

2. Cover and cook on low for 6 hours or on high for 3 hours, adding zucchini halfway through cooking. Season with salt and pepper

3. To serve, enjoy with couscous and yoghurt and sprinkled with coriander.

Cauliflower Korma

Time: 5 hours 10 minutes| Serving 4

Ingredients:

- 17 fl oz (500ml) vegetable liquid stock
- ½ cup tomato passata
- ¼ cup korma curry paste
- 2 ½ lbs (1.1 kg) cauliflower, outer leaves removed and base trimmed
- ⅓ cup Greek-style yoghurt, plus extra for serving
- ¼ cup pouring cream
- 2 tsp cornflour
- 1 deseeded and finely chopped tomato
- For serving:
- Long sliced green chilli
- Fresh coriander sprigs
- Toasted flaked almonds
- Roti, if desired

Preparation:

1. Mix together stock, passata and korma paste in slow cooker. Place the cauliflower upside down in the mixture and coat, stand it upright, cover and cook for 5 hours on low until tender, covered with the liquid

2. Mix together in a jug the yoghurt, cream and cornflour. Stir in to slow cooker and cook for 10 minutes to thicken the sauce

3. Serve cauliflower garnished with tomato coriander, chilli, and almonds. Serve with roti, if preferred.

Ratatouille

Time: 6 hours 20 minutes| Serving 6

Ingredients:

- 2 tbsp olive oil
- 2 garlic cloves
- 1 sliced red onion
- 2 large aubergines, in 1" (1½ cm) pieces
- 3 halved courgettes, 1" (2 cm) pieces
- 3 mixed peppers, 1" (2 cm)
- 1 tbsp tomato purée
- 6 chopped tomatoes,

- Small chopped bunch of basil
- Few thyme sprigs
- 14 oz can (400 g) plum tomatoes
- 1 tsp brown sugar
- 1 tbsp red wine vinegar
- sourdough, to serve (if desired)

Preparation:

1. Fry the onion in heated oil in a frying pan for 8 minutes. Add garlic and fry for 1 minute. Increase heat to medium-high, add aubergines and fry for 5 minutes until golden. Stir in courgettes and peppers, fry for 5 minutes until slightly soft

2. Add fresh tomatoes, tomato purée, herbs, canned tomatoes, sugar, vinegar, and salt and bring to boil. Relocate to cooker to cook on low for 5-6 hours

3. Season and scatter with basil. Serve with sourdough if desired.

Pasta e Fagioli

Time: 7 - 9 hours | Serving 6 - 8

Ingredients:

- ♦ 200g dried borlotti or cannellini beans, soaked for 6-8 hours
- ♦ 3 celery stalks, cut into chunks
- ♦ 2 carrots, cut into chunks
- ♦ 2 onions, cut into chunks
- ♦ 2 tbsp extra virgin olive oil
- ♦ 4 crushed garlic cloves,
- ♦ 34 fl oz (1 litre) vegetable stock
- ♦ 14 oz (400 g) can plum tomatoes
- ♦ 2 tbsp brown rice miso
- ♦ 4 bay leaves
- ♦ 6 rosemary sprigs
- ♦ ½ cup water
- ♦ 5 oz (150 g) ditalini rigati/small pasta
- ♦ 7 oz (200 g) cavolo nero with finely chopped stalks and torn leaves
- ♦ 1 oz (30 g) grated vegan parmesan, to serve

Preparation:

1. Bring drained beans to boil in salted water and cook for 10 minutes. After draining and rinsing, move to slow cooker, adding onions, celery and carrots. Stir in garlic, olive oil, stock, tomatoes, water and miso

2. Add herbs tied together with kitchen string. Season, cover and cook for 6 to 8 hours on low, until beans are cooked through and vegetables softened

3. Discard herbs, stir in pasta, cover and cook on high for 30 minutes. Add cavolo nero stalks and leaves. Cook for 30 to 40 minutes, until pasta is cooked through and greens tender

4. To serve, garnish with cheese and drizzle with olive oil.

Vegan Chilli

Time: 6 hours 15 minutes| Serving 4

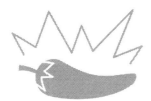

Ingredients:

- 2 sweet potatoes, peeled and cut into chunks
- 3 tbsp olive oil
- 2 tsp ground cumin
- 2 tsp smoked paprika
- 1 chopped onion
- 2 peeled and chopped carrots
- 2 chopped celery sticks
- 2 crushed garlic cloves
- 1-2 tsp chilli powder
- 1 red pepper, cut into chunks
- 1 tbsp tomato purée
- 1 tsp dried oregano
- 2 x 14 oz cans (400 g) chopped tomatoes
- 14 oz can (400 g) black beans, drained
- 14 oz can (400 g) kidney beans, drained

To serve:
- lime wedges, guacamole, coriander and rice

Preparation:

1. Cook onion, carrot and celery in heated oil in frying pan over medium heat for 8-10 minutes, stirring occasionally. Add crushed garlic and sweet potato chunks and cook for 1 minute. Add, oregano, all the dried spices, and tomato puree, cook for 1 minute and transfer to slow cooker

2. Add chopped tomatoes and red pepper, stir and cook on low for 5 hours. Stir in beans and cook for 30 minutes to1 hour

3. Season and serve with lime wedges, guacamole, coriander and rice

Breakfast Beans

Time: 5 hours 30 minutes| Serving4

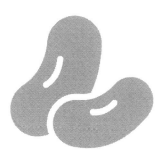

Ingredients:

- ♦ 1 tbsp olive oil
- ♦ 2 chopped garlic cloves
- ♦ 1 thinly sliced onion
- ♦ 1 tbsp soft brown sugar
- ♦ 1 tbsp white/red wine vinegar
- ♦ 14 oz (400 g) pinto can beans, drained and rinsed
- ♦ 6 ½ fl oz (200 ml) passata
- ♦ Small bunch coriander, chopped

Preparation:

1. Brown onion in a frying pan of heated oil, add garlic and cook for 1 minute. Add vinegar and sugar, and allow to bubble for 1 minute, before mixing in beans and passata. Season with black pepper and move to slow cooker

2. Cook on low for 5 hours. Stir in the coriander

3. Serve...

Sweet Potato Lentils

Time: 4 hours 55 minutes| Serving 6 - 8

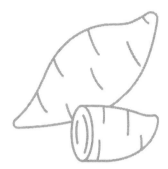

Ingredients:

♦ 3 cups vegetable broth

♦ 3 diced sweet potatoes

♦ 1 minced onion

♦ 4 minced garlic cloves

♦ 2 tsp garam masala

♦ 2tsp ground coriander

♦ 2 tsp chili powder

♦ salt

♦ 1 ½ cups uncooked red lentils

♦ 1 cup water

♦ 1can coconut milk

Preparation:

1. Cook vegetable broth, sweet potatoes, garlic, onion, and spices in cooker for 3 hours on high

2. Stir in lentils, cover and cook on high for a further 1 ½ hours.

3. Add coconut milk and water as needed. Stir

4. It is now ready to serve.

Chipotle Tacos

Time: 4 hours 20 minutes| Serving 4

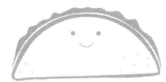

Ingredients:

♦ 2x 15 oz cans (425 g) pinto beans

♦ 3 oz (85 g) canned and chopped chipotle peppers in adobo sauce

♦ 1 cup canned corn

♦ ¾ cup chili Sauce

♦ 6 oz can (170 g) tomato paste

♦ 1 tbsp unsweetened cocoa powder

♦ ½ tsp cinnamon

♦ 1 tsp ground cumin

♦ 8 taco shells of your choice

♦ Toppings of your choice (lettuce, avocado, lime)

Preparation:

1. Place everything in slow cooker and cook for 3 to 4 hours on low or on high for 1½ to 2 hours

2. When cooked, spread a fair amount on the taco shells, topped with lettuce and any toppings of your choice.

3. Serve with beans and rice, if desired.

Disclaimer

This book contains opinions and ideas of the author and is meant to teach the reader informative and helpful knowledge while due care should be taken by the user in the application of the information provided. The instructions and strategies are possibly not right for every reader and there is no guarantee that they work for everyone. Using this book and implementing the information/recipes therein contained is explicitly your own responsibility and risk. This work with all its contents, does not guarantee correctness, completion, quality or correctness of the provided information. Misinformation or misprints cannot be completely eliminated.

Printed in Great Britain
by Amazon